THE CHEER DAD'S
SURVIVAL GUIDE

Cody H. Boyd & Stephen L. Koehn

ISBN: 9798325955754

DEDICATION

We would like to dedicate this survival guide to all the past, present, and future Cheer Dads. We appreciate your willingness to learn and hope this will help build more positive relationships with your athlete, their coaches, and the gym family as a whole.

CONTENTS

THE CHEER DAD'S SURVIVAL GUIDE

ACKNOWLEDGMENTS

Thank you to my wife Maggie. She is the hardest worker I know, and can take my ideas and harness me into action. Thank you to the Boyd family for trusting us with their cheer journey and Cody for being such a great friend and partner in writing this handbook. Lastly, to the entire staff at Flyer Athletics. Thank you for pouring your hearts into these athletes.

-Stephen

I have to start by thanking my awesome wife, Candice, and amazing daughter, Kiley. Their continued support for this guide, from concept to fruition, was instrumental in helping us build this as a potentially useful tool for Cheer Dads. I would also like to thank Stephen for his friendship and partnership in this endeavor. Finally, thank you to my fellow Cheer Dads and gym coaches, as their input was equally instrumental.

-Cody

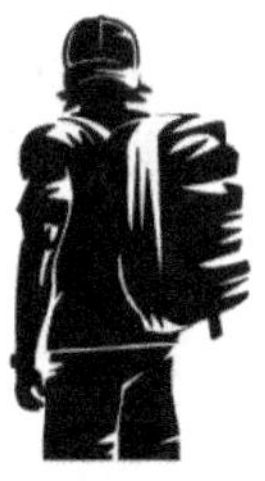

1 | INTRODUCTION

Competitive cheer is an amazing sport and one that neither of us thought we would be involved in as young men. That's the great thing about life and the way it pushes us into various directions, finding passions that we never knew we had.

The sport of competitive cheer, like many other sports, has a host of rules and regulations that we worked for years to understand. What is a double full or an arabian? Can a 12-year-old compete on a senior team? What does a score of 92 actually mean? If you have wondered about any of these types of questions, we are here to help!

Stephen is a current gym owner and coach at an emerging competitive cheer and dance gym in Tyler, Texas (Flyer Athletics). He is married to fellow gym owner and coach, Maggie, who spent years cheering professionally for the Indianapolis Colts and Houston Rockets after cheering for Baylor University. Stephen is the eternal optimist coach, who is very passionate about growing athletes professionally and personally.

Cody is a current Cheer Dad, whose daughter has been in the sport for about 10 years at various levels. Cody and his wife are active participants in their daughter's activities, including the cheer gym. They share a passion for competitive sports with their daughter and enjoy the growth and discipline opportunities offered through the sport of competitive cheer.

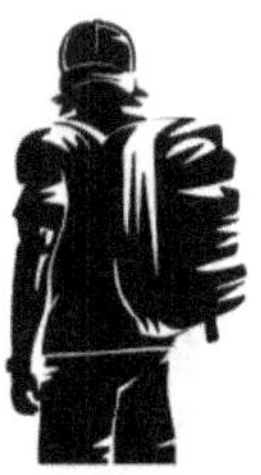

2 | COMPETITIVE CHEER EXPLAINED

Your athlete, son or daughter, has just joined competitive cheer and you aren't quite sure what you've gotten yourself into. It's a long road to know everything, but at the front of your thought is "What even is competitive cheer?" Well, welcome! This is perhaps this most loaded question in the history of cheerleading. First and foremost, competitive cheer is just that— competitive. It is also known as "All Star Cheer", so you will see that term used quite a bit.

If we look at the biggest college competition of the year, NCA 2024 in Daytona Florida, here were the results of one particular division. First place scored a 93.2056 while second place scored a 93.2042, on a scale of 0 – 100. We are looking at a difference of thousandths of a point. If you are new to the cheer world, don't worry. We will go over scoring later. However, this is one of the few sports that is decided by that thin of a margin. Competitive cheer is in fact, hyper competitive.

The second answer is competitive cheer is a commitment. It's a commitment to a team, to attempt to be perfect, and to oneself— that they can do hard things and achieve awesome results. It is a commitment to work as hard as you can, pushing through physical and mental battles for 10-12 months, only to perform for two and a half minutes. All Star Cheer is perhaps one of the biggest sport commitments throughout any age, from 3 years old to middle school, high school, college, and even professionally.

Lastly, you must know and understand that competitive cheer is a sport in its own world. Competitions can include over 1,500 cheer teams from all over the world. Arenas can pack in over 10,000 people, all screaming "1...3...5...7..." People will walk around spraying so much glitter that the air shines, and clothespins are legal currency. We have never experienced such lows. But we have never experienced such highs, either. Competitive cheer is without a doubt the hardest, most technical, and most rewarding sport there is.

As we go throughout this book, we will attempt to outline every little thing so that you are educated on the sport and can support your son or daughter the best way possible. But beware, all of us in competitive cheer are crazy. Regardless of that, welcome! We're glad you are here!

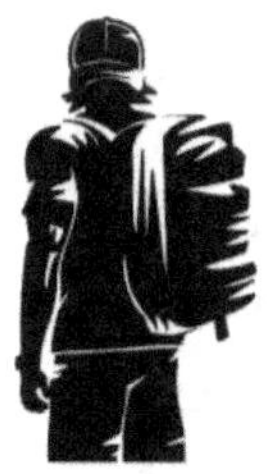

3 | THE BASICS

There are a few different types of teams in cheerleading that your athlete can be a part of. The most common three are novice team, prep team, and elite team. All three of these have various elements specific to them.

As far as scoring, it's just easier to say they are scored the same. In reality, novice teams have to do the least, prep teams have to do more than novice teams, and elite teams have to do the most. But all three follow similar score sheets. One more caveat is that novice teams are not given placements at competitions, instead they are given ratings (shown below).

Below 70% = Outstanding
71% - 84% = Excellent
85%+ = Superior

The biggest difference between these three types of teams is the length of the routine. Routine lengths are shown on the next page.

Novice: 1:30 routine
Prep: 2:00 routine
Elite: 2:30 routine

One of Stephen's biggest pet peeves is when people talk down to prep teams or novice teams because they aren't "elite." This is a common misconception. Regardless of whether your athlete is on a novice, prep, or elite team, they require a enormous amount of skill and dedication. Just because they may differ in routine duration or what their scoresheet looks like, it does not make any division easier than the other. It is just a classification of teams. As mentioned earlier, all competitive cheerleading is hyper competitive. If your athlete is on a Novice Level 1 team, they are just as much involved in All Star Cheer as an Elite Level 5 athlete.

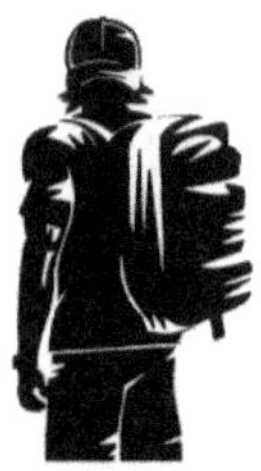

4 | TWO AND A HALF MINUTES

Alrighty, you're still here. That's awesome! We have welcomed you to All Star Cheer, and we have broken down the type of team your athlete may be on. Now let's talk about what they are doing in practice and what they will learn and perform.

Teams are scored on a few different aspects. This includes stunts, jumps, running tumbling, standing tumbling, toss, pyramid, and dance. We will dive a little deeper into the volume of these elements in our scoring section, but these are the seven substantive elements to Competitive Cheerleading. This is what they will be practicing for hours each week, in preparation of a competition. To learn all of this, they will be attending a lot of choreography sessions.

Choreography normally takes place late in the summer or early in the fall. As someone who is new to All Star Cheer, this can be a weird time because coaches will most likely ask your athlete to be at the gym from 8am - 8pm on a Saturday and Sunday for one weekend. It can be long and tedious. But this is where they learn their routine for the season. We will also note that, while the basic choreography is complete at this stage, your coaches will make adjustments throughout the year (based on judging feedback), to continually improve the overall performance and their score.

So, choreography is done, and they know their routine. Let's break down the seven elements.

- Stunts: These are some of the hardest and most technical elements of cheerleading. It is not an individual skill that can be worked on alone, as it takes a group of 2-5 people to make this work. Every athlete in the stunt has a very specific and very different job from the others in the group. Flyers must be extremely flexible and trust their group completely. Main bases (to the flyer's right side) must know every grip of a foot imaginable. Side bases (to the flyer's left side) must be smart and understand every possible outcome with the stunt. Back spots are the quarterback or point guard of the group. They must know everything and do everything all at once. All these athletes have to be extremely strong in their own right, or else the stunt fails. Stunts make up roughly 22% of a team's score.

- Jumps: This is where great athletes create separation from good athletes. In most routines, only the best athletes will jump, as jumps require extreme athleticism and perfect technique. There are three main goals in jumps: pointed toes, straight legs, and a tall chest. Height, while important and good when it's done correctly, does not matter if athletes cannot do those first the three. Jumps make up roughly 3% of a team's score.

- Tumbling: There is both standing tumbling and running tumbling in a routine, but they are each very different. Running tumbling is exactly what it sounds like, as athletes get a running start, so-to-speak. In standing tumbling, the athletes begin from a standing position. On a scoresheet (which we will talk about later), running tumbling is "cumulative", meaning tumbling passes are added up throughout the routine. Standing tumbling is different and must be done as a team, in sync with each other. Running tumbling and standing tumbling each account for about 20% of a team's score, so roughly 40% cumulatively.

- Toss: Whether you know a lot or nothing about cheerleading, you know a good basket toss when you see it. Similar to stunts, there is a group of 4-5 people, and their goal is to toss the flyer in the air. As simple as it sounds, it's not a simple skill. It is so hard to do this well. Flyers must be very confident in themselves and in their group, as they are possibly flipping and twisting in the air while the rest of the group prepares to catch them. Depending on the level that your athlete is on, certain air skills may or may not be permitted. For example, Level 1 cannot do basket tosses at all, as they are scored on a skill called a "show and go." Level 2 cannot twist, as it must be a "straight ride." Then it gets a little crazy from there. Tosses make up roughly 10% of a team's score.

- Pyramid: Arguably the fastest, most complex, most technical, and most fun to watch aspect of a routine is a team's pyramid. There is a lot that goes into this, but we will keep it simple. Think of this as all the stunt groups doing skills in sync, but doing all these skills while connected in a giant structure instead of individual stunt groups. What is so fun about pyramids is that teams get a chance to perform stunts that are a level higher than their current level. For example, a level 3 team can perform level 4 stunts in their pyramid since all the groups are connected. If you ever see coaches or parents closing their eyes, holding their breath, or crying during a routine, it's because their pyramid either hit perfectly or crumbled to the ground. A team's pyramid makes up roughly 22% of a team's score.

- Dance: Some athletes love dance, some athletes are indifferent, but every athlete must perform this dance perfectly. It must be in sync, with perfect formation changes, and be performed as big as it possibly can be. As a new Cheer Dad, you may be indifferent about this section, but nothing is more electric than a routine hitting perfectly and then the dance beginning! The team brings the energy, coaches are going insane, and the parents and fans are loving it. The dance makes up roughly 2% of a team's score.

All these elements together make up about 99% of the score. The missing 1% comes from an element on the scoresheet called, "Routine Mastery." This is where the performance comes into play. Is the spacing perfect? Is each athlete confident while performing? Is the team fun to watch? The only objective element here is the spacing and formations, so it's a tough one to see, but can be the difference between first and second place.

There are two reference charts in the back of the book. The first chart shows various elements of running and standing tumbling for levels 1-5. The second chart shows various elements of stunts for levels 1-5. These are not exhaustive lists and are only representative of some of the more basic aspects of each skill level. It's worth noting, that skills must be performed to counts and consistently, to benefit the routine. We are not going to attempt to define every skill as a lot goes into these elements, such as specific skills, creativity with transitions to different elements, and innovative formations. Our goal here is to outline a few of the main aspects that you will see in each level and the differences between them.

That covers the substance of a team's routine. So now we know what our team is doing, it's time to go compete and score high!

13

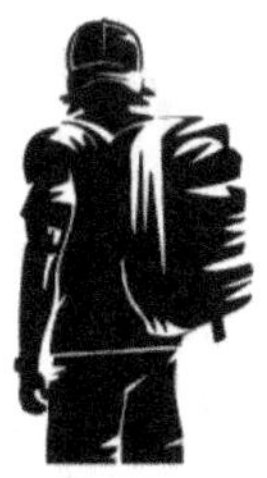

5 | CHEER ORGANIZATIONS

There are a wide variety of scoresheets used in All Star Cheer which can make this conversation confusing. However, most gyms attend competitions scored by one of these two. The Open Championship Scoring and United Scoring.

While most gyms compete on only one of these during their season, some gyms (like Flyer Athletics) compete on both. We can dive into why there are two score sheets later, but you need to understand scoring so that when your athlete comes off the floor and is waiting for their score, you can know exactly what needs to happen for them to potentially do well. If you really want to sound like a veteran Cheer Dad, start asking "What score sheet are we primarily competing on this season?"

The scoring conversation can get into the weeds quickly, so we are going to try and keep it short and sweet, giving you just enough information to know exactly what is happening in your athlete's routine. But we won't overload you where it keeps you up at night counting the number of tumblers that have to perform a particular tumbling pass. Cheer Dads need good sleep!

The Open Championship Scoresheet

There are many different competition organizations that use this scoresheet. This includes Redline, United, Bravo, and many more. All of these funnel into an end of the season event called The Allstar World Championships which takes place in late April. This scoresheet asks for teams to do a lot—and to do all of it well.

Stephen (as a coach and gym owner) finds this scoresheet to be very challenging. It asks for nearly every athlete on the team to do everything. This is a perfect example of why cheerleading is so difficult and competitive. In football you can have a player who primarily blocks, or who primarily runs the ball, etc. This particular scoresheet requires so much. It requires athletes to be versatile and good at every aspect of a routine, not just one particular element, for their team to score high.

The United Scoresheet

This scoresheet is what Varsity events use. Varsity is the "OG" of cheerleading, as it has now been around for over 50 years. Competitions such as Summit, Cheersport, and NCA use this scoring system. In our experience, this scoresheet is easier to attain certain "numbers." However, it is much more challenging in that this scoresheet demands perfection. If a routine does a lot but is not clean, it will undoubtedly score very low, on this scoresheet.

As a coach, Stephen believes that The United scoring system purposely asks for a little less to ensure that teams perform good, clean routines, though a lot must still be done. We have seen teams that have over-choreographed for this scoresheet in the hopes of outdoing other teams, only to be told the routine is not clean enough. Good, clean, high-quality cheerleading matters here more than anything. Athletes must be able to perform a skill with perfection.

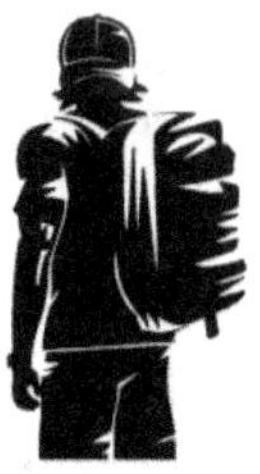

6 | SCORING OVERVIEW

Something you will hear coaches talk about a lot is "the numbers." Of all the things to understand about scoring, it is important to understand what your team has to do to score high. In football, we know that eleven players are on each side of the ball. Cheer is different, as teams can range from 5 - 38 athletes. Because of this, the score sheet asks different size teams to do different things. Why would a team of 5 do what a team of 38 does? So, the sport does a good job of making it clear for all teams.

In this numbers conversation, the words majority, most, max, and max+ (only on The Open Scoresheet) are used. Remember, we are not trying to get into the weeds here. Just know that you want your team to do the "max" number of tumbling, the "max" number of stunts and the "max+" number for their pyramid. If teams do this, they will max out the difficulty on their scoresheet. The difficulty is one of the few "objective" elements in cheerleading. If you do things by the numbers, you get that credit automatically on your scoresheet.

Almost all the remaining elements of the scoresheet are subjective. This is where it gets hard for parents and fans. You will find yourself asking why a particular skill was cleaner than another particular skill, and if a routine was "creative" and "innovative." Did your team do the bare minimum, as far as those numbers discussed earlier goes? Or did they go above and beyond? Was their technique good? These are all things for the judges to decide.

In Stephen's experience (as a coach) the winners of competitions using either scoring system, score a 96 or higher. However, we have been at competitions where a 95 (which is a pretty solid score), earned 11th place in a particular division and where a 93 won a different division.

The last thing you need to know about scoring before we wrap this up is that you always want your team to "Hit Zero". This means they had a routine with zero deductions. No one fell, there were no legalities or penalties, and there were no safety violations. Hitting zero is an awesome accomplishment! At the end of the day, we have seen and coached teams that have hit zero and lost and have seen and coached teams that have not hit zero and have won. So, hitting zero is the start to a good day, but the routine must still be hard enough and clean enough to earn a high score.

So after all that talk about scoring, what do you *really* need to know? Well, if your athlete's team scored in the 90's, they had a decent day and should be proud! If they scored 93-94, they had a good day! If they scored a 95, then now we can talk about winning! And if they scored a 96-97+...AWESOME! Let the placements fall where they fall, because a 96-97+ is an AMAZING day on any scoresheet.

Lastly, let's talk about winning. There are two ways you can "win" at a competition. The first is to win your division. This means that you are the highest scoring team within your age and skill level division. One example is if you are the winner of the Junior Level 3 Elite division. If you win your division, you have a chance to be a Grand Champion. Grand Champion means you are that competition's best team in your skill division, regardless of age. In the same example above, your athlete could win their division and then be the Grand Champion, meaning they beat out all other age divisions in their category. So, you have won your division, which is awesome. And you've won Grand, meaning you're the best elite team out of all levels at the competition! Some competitions award Grand Champion differently. It could be inclusive of all skill levels or broken down by level. Either way, winning Grand is a huge accomplishment!

In short, it's more than wins and losses, so always refer back to how your athlete's team scored and how their team is improving. But an absolutely perfect day would be something similar to scoring a 95+, winning your division, and winning Grand.

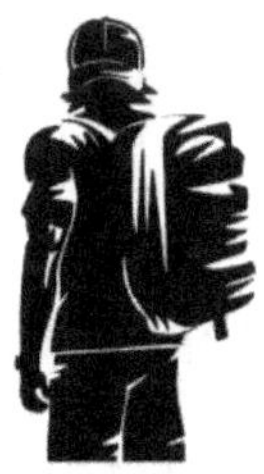

7 | AGES AND LEVELS

This is potentially the most glaring, confusing, frustrating, and talked about thing within the cheerleading world. So, let's set the record straight now. Your athlete's level does not matter. Read that again. Your athlete's level does not matter. Now, we obviously say that sarcastically as we all want athletes to strive for higher levels, set goals, and work hard to achieve them. But do not, we repeat, do not get bogged down in this conversation. If you can get in the right mindset, you will be off to a much more successful cheer season.

The first thing you need to know about is age groups, so let's break that down first. Age groups have nothing to do with levels. A Youth 2 team and a Junior 2 team are doing the same thing, literally. The only difference is the age. So, what age categories are there in all-star cheer? The age group categories are listed on the next page, with the approximate ages that are grouped into that category.

Tiny:	6-7 years old
Mini:	7-9 years old
Youth:	8-12 years old
Junior:	9-15 years old
Senior:	13-19 years old
Open:	18+

So, if you have a nine-year-old All Star Cheerleader, what age team can they be on? Well looking above, they can be on a mini team (7-9), a youth team (8-12), and a junior team (9-15). Which one is better? There is not a single correct answer here. However, in our experience it is better to keep the athletes with their own age groups as much as possible. Many parents will say their athlete does better with an older crowd, but this is just not the case. As a coach who creates teams year after year, we promise that gyms are doing their best to place your athlete where they will flourish! The success of the individual and the team is the priority, regardless of their age division.

Let's now address the biggest and most talked about concern (although it shouldn't be) of most All Star Cheer families in the springtime. "What level is my athlete going to be on?" We could write an entire book dedicated to this subject alone, but we won't. However, we will attempt to narrow this down to the three most important things that you need to know to be an informed Cheer Dad.

First, how many levels are there in cheer? There are seven (7) levels to All Star Cheerleading, although level 7 is reserved to only athletes 18+ years of age. Let's focus our efforts on levels 1-6. Therefore, there are 6 levels in All Star Cheer that your athlete can be on.

Now, remember that prep and elite conversation earlier (pgs. 7-8)? A lot of these levels have both a prep and elite level to them. Below is the breakdown of how the two work in terms of levels.

Prep Divisions	Level	Skills	Elite Divisions	Level	Skills
2:00 Routine	1.1	L1 Stunts L1 Tumbling	2:30 Routine	1	L1 Stunts & Tumbling
2:00 Routine	2.1	L2 Stunts L1 Tumbling	2:30 Routine	2	L2 Stunts & Tumbling
2:00 Routine	2.2	L2 Stunts L2 Tumbling	2:30 Routine	3	L3 Stunts & Tumbling
2:00 Routine	3.1	L3 Stunts L1 Tumbling	2:30 Routine	4.2*	L4 Stunts L2 Tumbling
2:00 Routine	3.2	L3 Stunts L2 Tumbling	2:30 Routine	4	L4 Stunts & Tumbling
			2:30 Routine	5	L5 Stunts & Tumbling
			2:30 Routine	6	L6 Stunts & Tumbling

Level 4.2 is an Elite team in its own right and is the outlier of the group.

This is a lot to take in at once, and we understand that. We also get that this may cause even more questions than it does answers. We will try to address that later. But for now, you need to know the difference and similarities between these levels.

Second, should my athlete move up annually, or at all? In short, no. As a Cheer Dad, you need to know that athletes must perfect a level before moving to the next level. There is no way around that. If a level is not perfected, the athlete should not move up. Go back to those elements to a routine (pgs. 10-12). If an athlete is not perfecting each of those elements, they should stay on that level until it is perfected.

This then begs the question, "How does my athlete get higher level skills if they are only competing on this particular level?" Good question. This is where tumbling classes and private lessons come into play. Team practices are focused on just that, the team.

An easy way to be an awesome Cheer Dad is to encourage your athlete to set goals that promote progress and to work to perfect where they are currently. In reality, athletes will not move up every year, athletes will not even move up every other year. Athletes may move up to a higher level one year and then move down to another level the next year. None of this truly matters. The only thing that matters is that your athlete is progressing in their skills and that you are at a gym that is putting them in a place to grow in their skills, physically and mentally, and succeed.

Lastly, does any of this truly matter? No. As we just mentioned there are only a few things that matter as far as the big picture is concerned in youth sports.

- Is your athlete improving, physically and mentally?
- Are they succeeding in their current position? Remember, success is not about wins and losses. Winning is only an aspect to being successful, not the entire definition of success.
- Finally, is your athlete enjoying their All Star Cheerleading experience? As a Cheer Dad, if you see these three things in your athlete, they are doing great!

Now, where all of this comes into play as a Cheer Dad is that you are better equipped to navigate these conversations with your athlete and spouse/partner. As a coach and as a Cheer Dad, we have both seen the good, bad, and ugly in terms of this level conversation. We hope you can discuss this in a sense that it is not always about moving up or being on a higher-level team year after year, but about succeeding where they are. The exhilaration of making a new level and the disappointment of not making it are very different dynamics. None of that matters. Help your athlete set very lofty goals! Then navigate your athlete in this conversation as they progress throughout the sport. This sport is great at developing athletes, but is even better at developing life and leadership skills that they will carry forward.

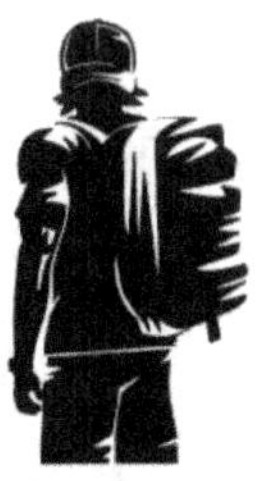

8 | WEEKEND SURVIVAL

As a Cheer Dad, surviving an All Star Cheer weekend requires a unique approach that balances support, involvement, and patience. Your role is crucial in providing the necessary encouragement and assistance to your cheerleader, and potentially your spouse/partner, while also managing the logistics and emotions that come with the intense competition atmosphere.

You will likely play a vital role in handling the logistics of the competition weekend, as well as offering emotional support. This includes organizing transportation to and from the venue, ensuring that your cheerleader has all the necessary uniforms, supplies and equipment, and managing the schedule to ensure that they are on time for all events. Plan ahead by purchasing your entry tickets ahead of time and booking a hotel close to or attached to the venue. Look at what parking is available, whether you will need to use a rideshare app, and the cost for each of these various items. Also, know the schedule. Most importantly, this includes knowing what time your athlete is due to report to their coach. This is usually hours before their actual performance time. By taking on these responsibilities, you can alleviate some of the stress and pressure on your cheerleader, allowing them to focus on their performance. This will also take some of the pressure off your significant other, which is an easy way to score brownie points!

Let's expand on the paragraph above for just a moment. Putting it bluntly, many dads are absent for cheer events. Cheer Dads are present and involved. It's important that you don't go into the weekend with few expectations of responsibility. Someone will need to pack the thousand items that go into a cheer weekend, make art out of hair, ensure the uniform is clean and pressed, perform makeup magic, make sure the athlete has food and water, pack the competition day backpack, etc. The morning of a competition can be very stressful, so it's important to be available and willing to offer a hand with whatever is needed. It is also beyond important to be patient. A report time of 7:00 am, will likely mean a wake up time of 4:30 or 5:00 am. Your Cheer Moms will be very appreciative of a Cheer Dad that is involved, supportive, helpful, and patient during a cheer weekend.

While supporting your cheerleader is a top priority, it's also essential to take care of yourself during the competition weekend. This is not always easy, as the food offered at most venues is nothing short of a diabetic coma. Plan ahead and see if the venue allows outside food. If so, pack some solid snacks, such as beef jerky, nuts, fruit, etc. If there is no food allowed in the venue, there is a well-known hack. Your bags may be searched for outside food, but your athlete's will not. It's funny how our athletes like the same food as us during these weekends! Also, be sure to get enough rest, and stay hydrated to ensure that you have the energy and stamina to keep up with the demands of the weekend. We are both big fans of caffeine and find that energy drinks and coffee are often foundational items for a successful cheer weekend! While you may be at a venue for many hours, your athlete will not be performing all day. Finding moments to relax and recharge can help you stay focused and present for your athlete when they need you most.

During the competition itself, be prepared for a rollercoaster of emotions as you watch your cheerleader perform. Stay positive and encouraging, regardless of the outcome, and offer constructive feedback and praise to help them grow and improve. Remember that your role as a Cheer Dad is to be a source of strength and support for your cheerleader, no matter what challenges they may face. Managing your own emotions and expectations is also crucial to surviving a competitive cheer competition weekend. It's natural to feel nervous, anxious, and proud all at once. But it's important to stay calm and composed for the sake of your athlete.

After the competition weekend is over, take the time to celebrate your cheerleader's achievements and reflect on the experience together. Win or lose, the bonds formed, and lessons learned during the weekend are invaluable. Use this time to connect with your cheerleader, share in their triumphs and disappointments, and show them that you are proud of their hard work and dedication.

By being present, organized, and supportive, you can help your cheerleader, and family, navigate the challenges of competition weekend with confidence and resilience. As a Cheer Dad, your role is not just to be a spectator, but a pillar of strength and encouragement, helping them achieve their goals and grow as a performer and individual. Also know that you are a part of team! Being present and supportive will make you want to be engaged and help, and the weekend will be much more fun.

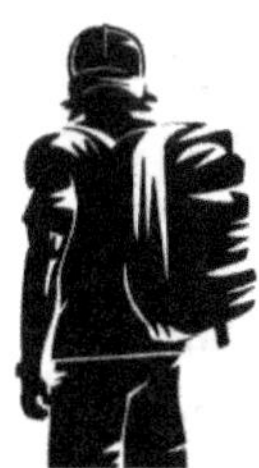

9 | THE IMPORTANCE OF FITNESS

Fitness is good for all of us, especially your All Star Cheerleader. We would both argue the amount of strength, power, endurance, and flexibility needed to compete at a high level is more than any other sport. What other sport requires you to flip your body, jump, and literally throw people in the air for two minutes and thirty seconds? Not one other sport. Don't let the hair and makeup fool you. This sport takes athleticism! So how do we get better at that?

First and foremost, be active. Any activity is a good thing. Walking together as a family in the evening, jumping on the trampoline, and playing with friends in the neighborhood are all simple and effective ways to be more active. This is good for all of us. It is that simple.

Second—resistance training. There is a giant misconception in the fitness world that resistance training for kids is a bad thing. Leave that mentality where it belongs, in the 1990's. If this is your mentality, we can confidently say that you are doing your athlete a disservice. We all know that males and females are created differently. But did you know that females are more likely to tear their ACL than males? There are a lot of studies that say different things, but all with the same theme, a lot of stress is put on athletes in this sport. Some studies say when athletes tumble, they are absorbing three times their body weight, and others say upwards of seventeen times their body weight. To decipher countless studies is not the goal here, but you need to know that your athlete's body is doing a high impact sport, and females are already at a disadvantage—with ACLs specifically. So how do we prevent injury? We get stronger.

How does your athlete get stronger? Well, just KIS. Keep! It! Simple! Body weight squats, lunges, and jumps of any kind are beneficial. Push-up and pull-up variations are always a great selection. If you have weights at home, awesome. Make your athlete use them! If you have a gym membership and your athlete is old enough for you to bring them, bring them! Make them do what you do. The reality is that your athlete will respond well to a wide variety of training so there is no need to overcomplicate this. The perfect program is the most practical program that works for you and your family. But we absolutely, highly suggest your athlete add resistance training into their routine, in some form or fashion.

Lastly, in terms of this fitness conversation and its importance in our sport, body image, self-esteem, and even ADHD can be greatly improved with exercise. We know this book is all about cheer, but the reality is that we know your athlete is busy beyond cheerleading. They may play other sports, do school cheer, clubs at school, or have a job. Exercise will not only help their cheerleading career but will help in literally every aspect of their life.

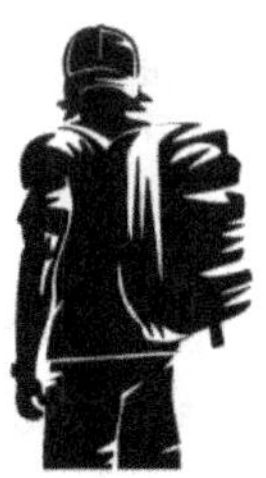

10 | YOUR CHEERLEADER

All Star Cheerleaders battle a lot. There is an insane demand from this sport on the athlete's time. Stephen, as a coach and gym owner, will admit that they ask a lot. This doesn't include school cheer, academics, friends, hormones, clubs, and just living the life of a kid or teenager. That being said, we will try to keep this to the point and highlight the greatest things to expect and be prepared for.

First, prepare for them to be frustrated. Remember, cheerleading is hyper-competitive and while you are battling other teams, the reality is that you are battling a scoresheet that demands perfection. We are all imperfect. We all know this. But it is our job to get these teams to score as high as they possibly can. That comes with the duty to work to achieve perfection with perfect technique, perfect timing, and perfect execution of all skills.

This demand for perfection will absolutely make your athlete frustrated. They will get in the car after practice and hate cheerleading. They will cry, be mad, and engage in every conceivable emotion. This is ok—we promise.

Now you do not want to be at a gym or in an atmosphere where this is an everyday thing, so please know that. Leaving practice daily feeling like this is in no way a good thing. The atmosphere all athletes should be in is one that is constantly encouraging and building them up. However, being frustrated absolutely comes with the sport. So be prepared.

Second, prepare for an emotional roller coaster. We do not mean your athlete directly. We mean that the sport is an emotional roller coaster in general. Your athlete will go to practice, learn, and accomplish a new skill, show up the next day, and not be able to do it. That is an emotional roller coaster. They will attend a two-day competition where they must qualify for Day 2, then they do not do their best—and that's a low. Then realize that they DID score high enough to qualify for Day 2—and that's a high! It's a roller coaster. Your athlete will work tirelessly for hours, for 10 months, then go to their end of the season event, do their very best, place high, then boom, it's all over. All that work for two and a half minutes, and then it's all over. That's an emotional roller coaster. Personally, we love this aspect of the sport. And we challenge athletes to embrace it. You should too. Nothing good comes easy. Take the good with the bad and enjoy the ride!

Third, prepare to watch your athlete learn to love their teammates unconditionally. This is such a cool aspect of our sport. The bond that it creates between people is unlike anything. Teammates must trust each other without fear. If a flyer is going to twist in the air, they must know and trust that their teammates will be underneath them no matter what. Athletes spend countless hours in the gym together striving for a common goal of perfection. That battle, day after day, hour after hour, forms this awesome bond between teammates. They see the good, the bad, and the ugly with their teammates. They celebrate their victories on and off the mat together. They are the shoulder to cry on when things get tough. And it's a team of people that are there for each other through it all. The life lessons of how to celebrate others when you may not be in the spotlight are invaluable. Learning to be empathetic, selfless, and proud of oneself are things this bond teaches that these athletes will be able to use for the rest of their lives.

Fourth, prepare for your athlete to fall in love with this sport. Call it crazy. Call it an addiction. Call it whatever you want. You'll see your athlete fall in love with competitive cheer like crazy.

All Star Cheerleading provides this crazy whirlwind of team success, individual success, highs and lows, winning and losing, blood, sweat, and tears. Rolled into hair, makeup, glitter, and literally screaming "1...3...5...7..." in an arena that has more people in it than your Friday night football game or your favorite college's sold out basketball stadium.

When first-time All Star Cheerleaders run out of the tunnel or up the ramp to take the mat for the first time, the feeling is overwhelming in the best way. That same feeling still happens to veteran athletes when they take the mat for the first competition of a new year. It happens every single competition. The whirlwind of emotion that has been built up from tryouts to summer workouts, to choreography, to now a competition, is unlike any other. You can't help but just fall in love with the atmosphere.

Lastly, prepare for *you* to fall in love with this sport. Expect to have more fun with your son or daughter than you ever had. Expect to travel and enjoy that time together as you wait in convention centers with them before they perform. Expect them to go through lows and be prepared to comfort them. Expect for them to have the highest of highs and be prepared to go crazy celebrating them. And never take a single extra practice, competition, or late-night car ride after practice for granted. Because at the end of the day this is time that you get with your son or daughter that cannot be replaced.

Most All Star Cheerleaders are involved in competitive cheer from grade 1 to grade 12. After that, it's gone. Cheer truly becomes a part of who your child is. By being present, it makes the sport a part of you and this is something you will always have together. Soak up all the time with your child that you can and love them through the sport that they love the most. We promise this sport will create memories that your child and your family will never forget.

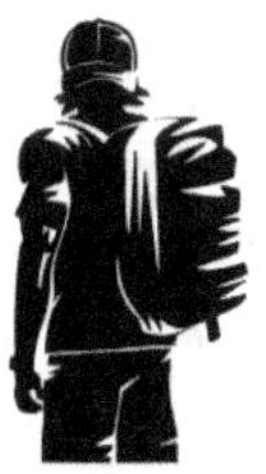

11 | A GOOD CHEER DAD

You have some of the basics down and you now know how you can help make your child a better cheerleader and teammate. But what about you? What can you do to be the absolute best cheer dad out there?

Your willingness to be involved is the perfect first step! However, being a good Cheer Dad is more than just showing up to your child's cheer competitions and practices. It involves being supportive, encouraging, and actively involved in your child's cheerleading journey.

As a Cheer Dad, you play an important role in helping your child succeed and thrive in this demanding sport. First and foremost, attend your child's cheer practices and competitions whenever possible. Your presence can make a big difference to your child and show them that you are invested in their cheerleading journey. It is important to show your support for your child's passion for cheerleading. A large number of dads rarely show up to any practices or competitions. They're missing out on a great opportunity to spend quality time with their child. Getting engaged and being a part of the team is the easiest way to get more comfortable with the sport, and even start to love it. Cheerleaders often perform better when they know their parents are watching and cheering them on.

One thing to note is that not all practices are open to the public. This means that the gym and team need some focused time to work on their routine, excluding any outside distractions. These are vitally important for any team's success. When you are allowed to attend practice, there are some simple rules of engagement to follow. This includes staying quiet and tucked away in the parent section of the gym. Also, just like any other sport, no one likes an armchair quarterback. Leave the coaching to the professionals. If you're reading this book, then you probably don't know enough to critique anyone! In the words of the great Nick Saban, "Trust the process.". Remember, the coaches are coaching a team, and not just your athlete.

Being a good Cheer Dad doesn't stop at the doors of the gym or convention center. Get involved in your child's cheerleading activities. Help with fundraisers, volunteer to help with organizing team trips, or even assist with what everyone is wearing to the events. By being actively involved in your child's cheerleading team, you show your child that you care about their interests and are willing to dedicate your time and energy to support them. If you have attended at least one competitive cheer event in your life, then you have likely seen a few groups of Cheer Dads, wearing dynamic and colorful outfits, walking in groups, and likely singing or listening to loud music. We aren't saying that you need to go to this extreme, but it does highlight the definition of "involvement" for some.

Competitive cheer is full of ups and downs. Your child will be working many hours to learn new skills, spending a lot of time on conditioning, and dealing with the dynamics of teams full of young kids and teenagers. Encourage your child to work hard and persevere in the face of challenges.

Cheerleading can be a tough sport that requires dedication, practice, and resilience. Remind your child that it is okay to make mistakes and that the important thing is to keep trying and improving.

It is not uncommon for an athlete to work for years to master a single skill. It involves some serious commitment and time on behalf of your kid. Celebrate these achievements, no matter how big or small. Whether your child masters a new stunt, wins a competition, or simply improves their skills, make sure to recognize and praise their hard work and dedication. Positive reinforcement can boost your child's confidence and motivate them to continue pushing themselves in cheerleading.

Be respectful to your child's coaches, teammates, and other parents. Cheerleading is a team sport that requires cooperation and teamwork. Your family will be spending a considerable amount of time with the rest of the gym family, so engaging positively will make life much more enjoyable. By modeling good sportsmanship and respect towards others, you also set a positive example for your child and help foster a supportive and inclusive cheer community. We have found some of our greatest life friendships are with people associated with the gym, and some of our most fun memories include these same people.

Finally, remember to have fun and enjoy the journey with your child. As mentioned above, cheerleading is a rewarding and exciting sport that can create lasting memories and friendships. Embrace the experience. Cheer loudly for your child. And savor every moment of their cheerleading journey. Be the Cheer Dad that is ok with jumping around with excitement and dancing when everyone is watching. If you woke up the day after a cheer weekend with no voice and sore muscles, then you've probably done your job.

REFERENCES

Tumbling: Running and Standing
*Not a complete list

LEVEL 1 SKILLS	
Running Tumbling Goal: 3 or more skills connected, without a pause—any variation.	Standing Tumbling Goal: 2 or more skills connected, without a pause—any variation.
Front Walkover - Cartwheel - Back Walkover	Back Extension Roll - Back Walkover
Cartwheel - Back Walkover - Back Walkover Switch	Valdez - Back Walkover
Round Off - Back Walkover - Back Walkover	Forward Roll - Forward Roll
Front Walkover - Round Off - Back Walkover	Back Walkover - Back Walkover Switch
LEVEL 2 SKILLS	
LEVEL 2 Running Tumbling Skills: 3 or more connected skills, without a pause.	LEVEL 2 Standing Tumbling Skills: 2 or more connected skills, without a pause.
Cartwheel - Round Off - Backhandspring	Back Walkover - Backhandspring
Front Walkover - Round Off - Backhandspring	Valdez - Backhandspring Stepout
Bounder - Round Off - Backhandspring	Back Extension Roll - 2 Backhandsprings
LEVEL 3 SKILLS	
LEVEL 3 Running Tumbling Skills: 2 connected level appropriate skills or any level appropriate skill connected by a lower level skill.	LEVEL 3 Standing Tumbling Skills: 3 or more connected skills, without a pause.
Front Walkover - Aerial	Standing 3 Back Handsprings
Front Walkover - Round Off - Back Handspring - Back Tuck	Jump - 2 Back Handsprings

Aerial - Chasse - Round Off - Back Handspring - Tuck	Back Handspring Stepout - 2 Back Handsprings
Punch Front - Round Off - Back Handspring Tuck	Back Walkover - Back Handspring - Jump - 2 Back Handsprings

LEVEL 4 SKILLS

LEVEL 4 Running Tumbling Skills	LEVEL 4 Standing Tumbling Skills
Punch Front Step Out - Round Off - Back Handspring - Layout	Back Walkover - Tuck
Round Off - Onodi - through to Layout	Jump - Back Handspring - Back Tuck
Front Handspring - Punch Front Step Out - through to Layout	Back Extension Roll - Back Tuck
Round Off - Back Handspring - Whip - Back Handspring - Layout	Back Handspring Step Out - Back Tuck

LEVEL 5 SKILLS

LEVEL 5 Running Tumbling Skills	LEVEL 5 Standing Tumbling Skills
Front Full	Jump - Back Handspring - Whip - Tuck
Punch Front Stepout - Round Off - Back Handspring - Full	Jump - Back Tuck

Stunts
*Not a complete list

LEVEL 1 STUNT SKILLS
Level 1 stunts require the backspot and the flyer to be connected hand to hand/arm for the duration of any single leg stunt
No inversions or tosses allowed
Quarter twisting is allowed
Stunts at extension must be on 2 feet

LEVEL 2 STUNT SKILLS
Inversions are allowed unlike Level 1
Baskets must be straight rides, no twisting in baskets
Half twisting is allowed
Stunts at extension must be on 2 feet

LEVEL 3 STUNT SKILLS
Coed stunts are allowed to single leg at extension
Baskets may involve twisting and other skills
Full twisting stunts are allowed
Stunts at extension can be on 1 foot

LEVEL 4 STUNT SKILLS
Inversions to extension are allowed
Full twisting releases to prep level are allowed
One and a half (1.5) twisting stunts are allowed
Releases from extension to prep are allowed (high-to-lows)

LEVEL 5 STUNT SKILLS
Release tik-toks at extension are allowed (high-to-high)
Switch kick full baskets are allowed (these are cool to watch)
1 ½ to extended single leg stunts are allowed
½ twisting stitch ups to extended body position are allowed

CHEER SEASON NOTES